I0075085

A Day In The Life Of An Ambulance Driver

The Good, The Bad and The Stupid

Adam Weddle

A Day in the Life of an Ambulance Driver

Copyright © 2016 by Adam Weddle

All rights reserved. No part of this book may be reproduced or transmitted in any form or by any means without written permission from the author, except in the case of brief quotations embodied in critical articles and reviews.

ISBN (978-0692823262)

Printed in USA

Dedication

This book is dedicated first and foremost to God. Without His favor and grace, this book would not been possible.

I also dedicate this book to both my mother, Jane, and my father, Phillip. They have been supportive of me my whole life. When I went to EMT school, when I decided to enter the US Navy they were there. It was them that encouraged me to go to paramedic school and continue to grow in this profession. Even from the onset of this book, they have been there.

My son, Zach, has supported and encouraged me throughout this process. He has had to sacrifice time together and he has given me many words of encouragement. It was also my desire to be a good role model and show him that we can do anything that we set our mind to.

I would also like to thank Ashley for all the support and encouragement that she gave me during the writing of this book.

Finally I need to thank Mary for the story that she told me so many years ago when I was lost for what I wanted to do in life. She is the spark that ignited the passion that I have had for this career.

Table of Contents

Introduction

A Day in the Life of an Ambulance Driver was born from the years that I have worked as an EMT and a paramedic. Over those many years I have been repeatedly asked to tell stories about my experiences. There have been so many experiences and stories over the years that it is always difficult for me to decide which one to tell when someone asks.

I have been asked which experience was the 'saddest', the 'funniest' or the 'hardest'. So I have tried to include a variety of stories within the pages of this book. They have all been told in the same way that I would tell them if I were telling it to you face-to-face.

In my youth I started keeping journals of life experiences. Some of those memories that I wanted to return to later in life just happened to be my experiences as an EMT. It has been those journals that have helped me to remember these experiences in such sharp detail.

Most of these stories are directly from my personal

experiences. However there is one that is obviously not mine, but it was instrumental in my decision to go into this line of work. That story has been relayed as closely to the way she told it to me as best as I could recall. Also there are a couple of others that I have included as though they were mine, but were in fact experiences that were told to me in great detail by close friends. They were kept in the same tone as the rest to help mask the identity of those involved.

Finally I have intentionally left out some of the details, such as specific cities, race/nationality, etc. in an attempt to help protect the identities of the patients that I have had the pleasure to treat. If you had been in the position of some of my patients, I am sure you would not want your identity exposed either.

I dearly hope that you enjoy reading these stories as much as I have enjoyed writing them.

Fleas, Fleas, Fleas

This is the story told to me by a friend when I was in high school which made me want to become an EMT. She was one of my neighbors at the time and had been an EMT for several years before she got married. There are going to be many of you that will scratch your head and ask why on earth this story would pique my interest in this kind of work. Stick with me until the end and I will explain it all to you.

It was a nice summer day and we were sitting on the porch talking. It was me, my mom and sister and Mary. She occasionally would talk about some of the weird things that went on while she was an EMT. At the time, I was going into my senior year of high school and had no idea what I wanted to do for a career anymore. For as long as I could remember, I had always wanted to be an architect, but after going through a couple of drafting classes that just no longer interested me.

Mary started talking about a day when she and her partner were dispatched to pick up a patient to take to hospice care. For those that are not familiar, hospice is for people that are terminally ill and want to only receive comfort care instead of the all-out life-saving treatments. She went on to explain how the house was in a part of town that no one went into after dark. The houses were not in the best kept conditions and very few if any had air conditioning. Most of them were lucky if they could afford a fan to stir the air.

When they arrived at the home, they were greeted by the patient's family. It was one of the patient's children that had chosen to take care of their father in his final years. They were told that he was in a bedroom on the first floor of the house. Fortunately there were only two steps going up to the porch. She went on to describe the house as being swelteringly hot and smelled of ammonia from the uncleaned cat litter boxes that were in several places in the house. Sadly this is not an unfamiliar situation for those that have worked in EMS for very long.

She told us that when they walked into the bedroom they found their patient lying on a few blankets on the floor. He was definitely not in very good health and had not been very well taken care of.

The added smell of sweat and urine made it all the more unbearable. So they looked at each other, and knowing each other as well as partners tend to, they nodded in agreement that they needed to do a fast load onto the cot and get the heck out of there.

They lowered the cot as close to the floor as they could and opened all the buckles. Mary, as it was her turn to be the patient tech, assessed the patient as she explained to him what they were going to do. She remembered rather vividly that he was not really in a very alert state, but she didn't know if that was his normal state because of his illness or if it was because of the lack of care he was obviously getting. After doing a very brief look over, she said she was ready to move him to the cot. Vital signs would be taken in the ambulance, as it had air conditioning.

Mary assumed her position at his legs and her partner at his head. Mary was to grab under his knees while her partner would lift from under the man's arms so that they could lift him up to the cot. As they both reached under him, they both jumped up in shock. There was a swarm of bugs that scattered from under each place they had just placed their hands. After they took a quick second to compose themselves, they had looked closer and saw that they were fleas. Fleas were now crawling all over the patient and the floor and both of them.

They each did the best they could to brush the fleas off them and after a very quick discussion, decided that it was best to get this man out of this house and they would deal the best they could with these fleas. Each of them grabbed a towel and they rolled him onto his side to try to brush away as much of the infestation as they could. Fleas swarmed from under this poor man's neck, lower back, under each knee and armpit. The exposed areas in each of these spots was red and swollen from the constant biting of these pests. The partners did their best to get as many of them off of the patient as possible and quickly secured him to the cot and got the hell out of dodge.

After they got into the truck, Mary told her partner to just go and drive fast. She was doing her best to deal with the fleas and the patient while she had shivers crawling up and down her back thinking about the bugs crawling on her.

The ambulance was cruising down the highway when the rain started to come down pretty hard. Mary felt her partner start to pull to the side of the road, but before she could ask why, her partner was yelling for her to come up to the cab. When she got up there, she heard this awful screeching noise coming from the windshield. Her partner then told her that the driver's side wiper blade had fallen off and she couldn't see because the rain was coming down so hard. She asked if she should call dispatch and have them send another truck or at least someone with a new blade. Mary said that she may have muttered a few expletives before saying that she wasn't going to be stuck in the back of that truck with all the fleas nibbling on her while they waited for another truck. So she told her partner to hold on. She then ran out in the rain and grabbed the blade from the passenger side of the truck and moved it to the driver's side. Then she put a couple of 4x4s under the empty arm on the passenger's side to hopefully keep it from scratching the window. It seemed to work, she told us, so they started back down the highway towards the hospice facility, albeit at a slower pace.

Mary explained that she didn't want to surprise the staff with the bugs that they were dealing with, so she made a quick call on the radio to let them know. The nurse told her that they could not accept a patient with fleas. They had no way of dealing with that kind of problem and they would need to divert to the county hospital. This was obviously NOT what she wanted to hear. She told her partner to turn around and head to the county hospital.

She then called them on the radio to tell them of the situation and they told her that they would be ready for her on arrival. She explained that at the time, she didn't know what that meant. As they pulled into the ambulance bay, they were met by people in big white hazmat suits. A few of them took the patient to one part of the bay that was curtained off and then a couple of others took her and her partner to another area. They were ushered into a make-shift shower area and told that they needed to completely disrobe and scrub down with some special soap. She said looking back, it feels a little embarrassing, but at the time she was just happy to be getting all those creepy crawly bugs off of her skin. They were given towels and a clean pair of scrubs to wear home. Needless to say that was the end of that shift for both of them.

She said that later they were told by the supervisor that the people at the hospital had bombed the ambulance with pesticide to kill all the fleas and that every piece of equipment had to be cleaned and every supply replaced. She said that as they were taking all of the contaminated stuff off they were finding that fleas had even gotten into the sterile, sealed packs of equipment. Fleas are nasty little bugs.

For months after this incident, she told us, her co-workers would put flea collars and flea powder in her and her partner's lockers. There was a lot of good-humored jokes made. She said that even on occasion years later, she would get a random flea collar in the mail from someone.

As I said at the beginning, many of you are probably scratching various parts of your body as you feel imaginary fleas crawling on you, and asking why on God's green earth would this make me want to become an EMT. Well, while I definitely do not want to recreate this event for myself, it spoke of adventure, humor and a close camaraderie that I wanted to be a regular part of my life. Even though this could have very well been a traumatic event for many of you reading this, Mary told us this with a smile and several bursts of laughter. I have always loved telling stories, as you may deduce from my writing of this book, and this kind of life fit in with my personality. I have had many adventures of my own as you will read in the coming pages and I have never regretted my decision to join the ranks of the Emergency Medical Profession.

My First Lesson

I will forever remember my very first run on an actual ambulance. Not because it was gory or bad, but because I learned a valuable lesson and it was extremely exciting finally getting to ride in a truck that was floating down the street with lights and sirens on.

We, the students, were all scheduled to ride out on the ambulance at a local fire station. On my first day, a sunny Sunday, at the fire house we were having a fairly slow day and I was mostly enjoying talking to the firefighters about their jobs and checking out all the trucks. It was in the early afternoon when the first call for an ambulance came in. The tones in the fire station rang throughout the whole building. My heart immediately started to beat faster as I listened to the dispatcher give the details of the call, the address and the nature of the distress. We were being sent to assist an 'unconscious person'.

I climbed in the back of the big rig, which is where the students were always supposed to ride. First the engine pulled out and then we filed in line right behind them. It wasn't far, just a few turns and we were arriving on the scene. It was now that I, as the excited student got to do my duty. I got to carry the bags to the patient. A couple of the other firefighters lagged behind to pull the cot from the rear and bring it to us.

The on-duty paramedic and his EMT partner rushed into action as they quickly approached the man who was lying on his back in the middle of the front yard of the home we were called to. From a quick glance, he looked to be possibly in his mid-40s and he looked to be somewhat sweaty and maybe a little pale. There was a lawn mower not too far from him. So the medic was going in to make the assessment. Did he get too hot while mowing the lawn and have heat stroke or exhaustion? Possibly the strain of yard work caused him to have a heart attack? Or maybe he was experiencing some other medical condition that had nothing to do with the immediate environment, such as seizures or cancer?

Of course the first thing every good EMT and medic do is assess and secure a patent airway and check for a pulse. So the EMT immediately grabbed the patients head and started to do a jaw thrust to open the air passage in the throat. The paramedic went into action removing the patient's shirt to expose his chest for the heart monitor. However, this is where things got a little hairy.

The patient was not actually unconscious!!!

As it turns out he had in fact been doing some yard work and did get hot and tired. So he decided to lie down under his tree for a rest and apparently ended up taking a small nap. Let me tell you that I was never so happy to be the STUDENT this time and not the person that was abruptly waking this man from a nice afternoon nap. There were a few expletives shouted and I think a half awake kind of punch thrown. Fortunately no one was injured.

The odd thing about it was that this poor guy was not the slightest bit awakened by the sound of sirens and big diesel engines pulling up to the front of his home. He must have been pretty tired or a very sound sleeper.

It was a great first run to begin my career as I learned a very valuable lesson that I have carried with me throughout my whole life. Always start a patient contact by speaking to the potential patient and then checking for responsiveness with some gentle touch before grabbing someone's face and attempting to disrobe them.

I Almost Didn't Make It

Growing up I had seen a fair amount of blood and it never really bothered me. During high school a friend and I watched every single episode of the Faces of Death movies. Whether it was in person or on TV, I never was really effected by blood or death. That is why I was a bit surprised at my first patient experience during EMT school.

One of the clinical rotations was in the emergency room shadowing a nurse. The ER in the hospital that I was going to EMT school was a level 1 trauma center. That means that they got it all, from stubbed toes to gun shots and car accidents. After my assigned nurse gave me the tour of the ER, she went into a room with an elderly patient that had fallen and split her scalp open on a table. The bleeding had mostly stopped by the time we went in to start assessing her vital signs and the injury, but it was going to need stitches. After the doctor finished his exam, he asked the nurse to set up a suture kit. I wanted to watch this because I had never watched how sutures were placed.

As the doctor was getting ready to start numbing up the area, I really started to notice an odd smell in the room. This smell was not like any blood smell that I had ever experienced before, but then again I don't remember ever being in a closed room with someone that was bleeding either. Never-the-less I sat and watched with rapt attention as he started to clean the wound up.

The longer I sat in the room and watched the more I was getting a feeling like I was going to vomit. Not wanting to throw up in front of the patient, or the staff, I excused myself out of the room. Surely vomiting while watching someone get stitches was not a reason to kick someone out of EMT school, but I didn't want to take the chance. Sitting at the nurses station, I was feeling pretty embarrassed that I could not handle a little blood. It made me start to question if I would be able to handle something major, like an amputation once I got into the field. Fortunately I did not have to sit and stew very long before the nurse emerged from the room.

"Wow! The alcohol smell got pretty thick in there? I almost couldn't take much more either." she said as she walked towards me. She sat down to finish documenting her patient care for the poor elderly woman and told me that the patient had drank a bottle of vodka tonight and that was what had caused her to fall.

Whew! I had not realized that the old lady had been drinking and had never been around someone that drunk to know what it smelled like. It was a tremendous relief to know that it was not blood that was making me queasy.

They tried to admit the woman for overnight observation because a head injury in an alcoholic can be deadly if she started to bleed into her skull later. However this woman was not going to have any part of being made to stay in a hospital. I guess it probably had to do with the fact that they would not let her drink. To each their own!

Sex With A Diabetic

Today there are bariatric beds in almost every hospital. Ambulances have access to cots that can handle up to 1200 lbs. We have gotten to a place in today's society that being grossly over-weight has become commonplace and accepted. This next story took place before that was a truism.

It was a late fall evening and I was a fresh EMT riding with my favorite crew on the local 911 ambulance. We got dispatched for an 'unconscious person'. We arrived at a little old house on a dimly lit street in a poorer part of town. We went to the front door of the house and knocked. A very tall, probably 6'5"-6'6", very skinny black man answered the door. He invited us inside the home and explained that he called 911 for his wife. As he led us back to the bedroom where she was he explained what was going on. It seems that he and his wife had been having sex and at one point he noticed that her eyes rolled up and initially he assumed that she was having an orgasm. However when she never came back around, he became concerned as she was just recently diagnosed with diabetes and called 911. As we rounded the corner into the bedroom he finished up with the fact that she has not been ambulatory (able to walk) for over 6 months now.

What we saw next took us all a little aback. As we entered through the bedroom door, we observed a very obese woman lying on a mattress that was on the floor. To give everyone an idea of just how shocking this was, at the hospital she weighed in at over 800 lbs. As you can probably guess, not having walked in over six months, this patient has been using the bathroom and bathing in this bed for at least that long. There was a somewhat dank odor that hit our noses as we approached her to begin assessing her. We all looked at each other with a knowing glance as we all realized that her husband had also just said that they were just having sex.

The medics tried to arouse her and she would moan and kind of open her eyes but was not really responsive. One medic began placing the heart monitor on her as the other began getting the IV equipment ready. They started an IV and checked her blood sugar with was registering only as "LOW". Therefore they administered some glucose (sugar) through the IV and she almost immediately became more alert. Due to the recent diagnosis of diabetes and the episode of a severe low blood sugar, the medics recommended that she be transported to the hospital for evaluation. She and her husband agreed.

The fire engine was on-scene with us and began to evaluate how to 'extricate' the patient from her home into the ambulance. The officer on the truck called for a tactical unit so that they could cut a portion out of the bedroom wall leading to the outside to move her. Upon hearing this dispatch, the battalion chief came to see what was going on. While the fire guys were discussing what needed to be done to cut the wall out, the chief stepped in and said that these people were poor and would not be able to afford to fix an exterior wall before winter. He said that there was no need to cut a hole in the wall because, "it's just fat, it squeezes". Everyone chuckled, but knew that he was probably right.

Two of the firefighters were tasked with putting

the ambulance cot on top of the fire engine and removing all the hardware from the floor of the ambulance. The rest of us took a heavy tarp into the bedroom and laid it out on the floor next to the bed. Since the patient was alert, the medics asked her to roll herself onto the tarp. She needed assistance from a few of the guys though. While I believe that most of the people reading this probably would feel completely embarrassed by having to go through the ordeal of 'rolling' onto a tarp to be taken out of their house; this lady was laughing and saying, 'weeee' as she was rolled over and over.

There were four of us on each side of the tarp and on person at the foot and one at the head. We moved her over to the door of the bedroom and then a few guys went into the hall as we began the process of squeezing her through the door. As the chief suggested, she did in fact squeeze through. Then we all got back onto the tarp and moved through the house and did the process again at the front door. Once we got her to the ambulance, a few other firefighters joined in and climbed into the back of the ambulance and we all managed to lift her onto the floor of the back.

The transport was uneventful and the medic just did his report and called in to the hospital so that they could obtain a bed that was able to handle the weight of the patient. As we arrived, the ER staff was waiting in the bay with the bed at the ready. That made it much easier as we rolled the bed up to the end of the ambulance and simply slid her out onto it.

I think that the visual that has most stuck in my head over all of these years is after the hospital staff removed the patient's nightgown. Both of her breasts were laying on the bed at her side and her belly extended down almost past her knees. The thought returned to all of us that the husband had told us that they had just been having sex. We didn't even want to attempt to figure out those logistics.

In concluding this story, I want to add a personal after thought. Over the years I have had the experience of hearing smokers and extremely obese people say that they can live their life the way that they choose and everyone else needs to butt out and mind their own business. Maybe you have felt this way or have known someone that does. However what has been my experience is that after these people have gotten to live their life the way they want, they expect those of us in the medical field to clean up their mess. We have to strain our backs lifting the obese that got to eat all they wanted. We are expected to be compassionate and understanding when a smoker gets cancer or COPD and feels like they are drowning everyday of their life. It all of a sudden becomes our burden to take away their pain and save their life more frequently than the normal patient due to the consequences of their poor life choices. So please keep in mind that the choices that you make today will likely have consequences later in your life, some good and some bad. So when the bad consequences happen, remember that the people that are taking care of you are doing it out of a compassionate heart because they didn't force you to do the things that make you sick. Rant over!

Happy New Years To Me

Many years ago, when I was a young man and still considerably shy when it came to girls, I had the fortune to respond to a minor car crash on the early morning of New Year's Eve going into New Year's Day. The car that my ambulance was directed to was occupied by three Hooters waitresses on their way home from a long night of work and had gotten hit by a drunk driver. It was still unseasonably warm for this time of year and it had just finished raining. These girls were all still in their uniforms since it was not cold.

Our crew consisted of two paramedics and me as the EMT. We took two of the girls as our patients and placed them both on back boards with the assistance of the firefighters and loaded them into our ambulance. The girls' injuries were minor, mostly scrapes from broken glass and a few bruises, and we were primarily taking them to the ER to just be checked out to make sure that there were no internal injuries that we could not find. The firefighters carried one girl to the ambulance where she was secured to the bench seat.

One of the medics took over care for her and began to assess her. The other girl was placed on the cot and she was my patient.

Since there was not much to do after our initial assessment, the ride was pretty boring. The paramedic was mostly writing his run report and calling into the hospital to let them know what we were bringing them.

The next part of this story was a little embarrassing for me to say the least. At that time, I had not had many dates and was still starry eyed when it came to the ladies. As both of these girls were in the skimpy uniform that Hooters' girls wear, I was apparently in awe of the chest of the girl on the bench seat. She looked over at me and took notice of my staring and she politely grabbed my attention and asked for a blanket. Just to show you how smooth I was, I quickly grabbed the attention of the medic and told him that her 'respiratory rate' was 20 and then started to take her blood pressure. I'm quite sure that she didn't buy it as my face was a burning bright shade of red.

The rest of the trip was uneventful. However when

we arrived at the emergency room, I took my patient to the assigned room and helped move her to the bed. She was noticeably scared and she asked if I could stay and try to call her dad to tell him where she was. I agreed eagerly. After not being able to reach him, she asked if I could stay with her because she was scared. Today, I would assure her that she was in great hands and they would send someone in to help her reach her father while I had to go out to help others. However, then was not 'today'. In my young naive state, I thought that maybe I had a chance to date this beautiful young woman and maybe even get a girlfriend. So I stayed after letting the other guys know that I was not going back out with them. (P.S. I was just doing a ride along, not getting paid. Therefore I didn't leave my job for this.)

I ended up staying for several hours by her side holding her hand and reassuring her that everything was going to be OK. After all the testing was done, it was determined that she had not sustained any major injury and would be released after just a few hours of observation. In the early hours of the morning, her father did finally arrive. It was at that time that I did finally leave and asked for her number to 'check in' on her later, which she gladly gave me.

In the weeks that followed, I did eventually realize as I continued to pursue a date with this girl, that I was being put off and she was starting to get a little bored with my lack of being able to 'get the hint'. In hindsight, I do see how annoying I probably was and I learned that many times a scared patient will latch onto her first responder.

My Belly Is Hurting

Please understand as you read this story and many others throughout this book, that many of us in the emergency medical field (EMTs, nurses and doctors) tend to either have or develop a sort of twisted sense of humor about the things we see and in the way we react to some situations. Where some will see sorrow, tragedy and have sympathy, we tend to find humor and stupidity. Try not to judge us as you read the words that follow.

During my 20s, I was a corpsman in the U.S. Navy. By far some of the best times in my life. However during my tenure at one of the naval hospital emergency departments, I got to witness some rather funny things that people do. This probably was partly due to the fact that I worked the overnight shift most of the time. Partly because when people get drunk and think when they do stupid things under the shadow of night that it will be OK.

NEVER DO ANYTHING THAT YOU DON'T WANT

TO HAVE TO EXPLAIN TO A PARAMEDIC!

It was a late Friday night and this young military man walked into the emergency department waiting room. He approached the check-in desk and explained that he was having severe abdominal pain and needed to see a doctor. Patients never want to tell the people up front all the stupid things that they do, so they come up with some mundane, albeit real, symptom to get in the back to see a doctor. This young man was in obvious pain and was having trouble sitting still. At this point, the ER had not gotten too busy yet, so we put him on the top of the stack of patients and took him back to a room fairly quickly. Anyone that has experienced severe stomach cramps understands that curling up laying on your side helps, instead of sitting on an uncomfortable seat in a waiting room.

He was put in a bed in my area of the ER, so I was responsible for helping get him checked in and get his vital signs and changing him into a gown. While I was doing all of this, the doctor had come in and started his evaluation of the patient. During the part of the exam where the doctor was asking when the pain started, the patient started talking in a very low, almost inaudible tone. After being told to speak up so the doctor could hear him, we listened as he explained that he had purchased a vibrator. It was the kind that the tip was curved and, when turned on, rotated in a circular motion. Of course, in his embarrassment of having to explain this to someone, it took this poor boy far longer to get all of that out of his mouth. He went on to explain how he was using it on himself while masturbating and apparently the circular motions caused it to 'crawl' up into his rectum to a point that he could not reach it. He went on to explain through choked back tears that he tried to push it out on the toilet and dig in with his fingers but it just kept getting farther up inside of him and eventually caused him a lot of pain.

Some of you are probably reading this and feeling truly sorry for this young man and the predicament that he was in. However, the doctor and I, were having a very hard time keeping ourselves from laughing at him. Unfortunately I think it showed. In the most professional tone that the doctor could muster, he explained that he would have to get x-rays and consult with a surgeon to figure out what they needed to do.

Before I get any further into this, please keep in mind that this is all taking place before it was in any way acceptable for a gay male or female to be in the military. I have no way to say whether this particular person was gay or not (I understand that some straight males do enjoy things in the butt), the implication of having a dildo stuck inside of you, as a man, was enough to create at least some doubt as to what you were.

After getting all the needed tests, the surgeon came in to talk with the boy. Not wanting to miss out on anything, since I would be the person prepping the patient if he were to go to surgery that night, I followed the doctor in and took some vital signs while listening in. The surgeon explained that he looked at the x-rays and that indeed the vibrator had maneuvered its way deeply into the patient's colon. He went on to say that surgery was going to be needed, but that he needed to know one thing before he could proceed with the prep.

These are the words that the surgeon said and they will forever ring in my memory. "Son, you understand that we will need to go into surgery to fix this problem." To which the young man shook his head in the affirmative. "But before we go in there, I need to know one thing... Do you want us to remove the thing, or just replace the batteries?"

The surgeon and I were literally on the verge of an unprofessional burst of laughter. The boy on the other hand burst out in tears and rolled over. Part of me felt so bad for him and the fact that, in the military, we all lose a little bit of our normal rights to dignity and professionalism. This kind of statement would never have been even the slightest bit acceptable in the civilian world, but in ours it was a part of the culture.

Ultimately, he went to surgery and they simply went up his colon and removed the apparatus and he went home in the morning physically no worse for the wear. I did hear that after they removed it, they did ask if he wanted it back but he declined and told them to please throw it in the trash.

We Are Lifesavers

The lesson to be learned from the following story is: If you don't want EMS to do anything, then do NOT call 911!

As a newly graduated and state certified EMT, I was probably a little bit overly gung-ho. With the help of an awesome EMT instructor, I was able to put together a medical 'tech' bag that made the one on the ambulance look like a purse. Yes I was a volunteer firefighter with too much enthusiasm.

Our fire station was dispatched with the local 911 medic on a possible cardiac arrest. I was pretty close to the dispatched address, so I was the first to arrive. I grabbed my tech bag out of my trunk and ran, head first, into the home. In retrospect, I think that I thought I was going to be the lone hero that saved the day.

Upon getting inside, I was led to an older lady in a bed in the middle of the living room. She was being attended too by a home healthcare aid who was the person that called 911. As I approached the patient to begin my assessment, the aid began quietly telling me that 'It's okay, she is dead.' Stunned I was halted in my tracks and I asked her to repeat what she said. 'She has MS and she is dead, so it's okay. I just need you to take her body away.' It only took a few seconds for me to process what she said, to which I responded, 'Then you shouldn't have called 911. We are legally bound to try to save the patient.'

I went to work (while ignoring the aid) on opening the patient's airway and checking for breathing. There was none. I checked for a pulse. There was none. However she was warm and still pink in color. That meant that she had not been 'DEAD' for very long. So I opened my back and got out a Bag Valve Mask (BVM) and started to give her a couple of breaths. As I was beginning to breathe for her, the medic crew walked in with a couple other volunteers and they started compressions and hooking up the heart monitor. She was indeed in V-fib, a lethal heart rhythm. So we quickly loaded her up onto the cot and headed for the ambulance while doing CPR.

In the back of the truck I took over doing

compressions while the paramedics delivered shocks to the patient's heart and started an IV. One of the other firefighters started to drive us to the hospital. As an EMT, all I could really do was basic CPR, so I stuck with doing chest compressions to let the medics do the advanced stuff. As we got close to the emergency room, one of the paramedics announced that we got a sinus rhythm back. The other checked for a pulse and stated that she had a good one. We pulled into the ambulance bay and took the patient into the ER and handed off care to the doctor and staff.

This was the first time that I had actually had a part in saving a life. It was an amazing feeling. The doctor even came out after they had stabilized the patient and told us what a great job we did. This run made a significant impact on my life going forward and hooked me on working in EMS. However I would like to say that while we did our duty and did it well, there are times when there is a little doubt in the back of my mind if we did the 'right' thing for this patient. She was bed bound and for all outward appearances non-communicable with the world she lived in. Maybe she would have been better off if we had let her pass in peace. In the end though, that was not and is not my call.

Just Like A Movie

It was early evening when the call came in over the pager for the volunteer fire department where I was working. The dispatch was to an address that was right around the corner from my home so I knew that I needed to go. The dispatch came out as a possible DOA (Dead On Arrival). As it turned out the police were sent to this address earlier to check on the person that lived there.

I was still a new EMT and had not yet seen a dead body in person. That is probably more of the reason that I went than the fact that I was close. I got there about the same time as one of the more seasoned EMTs on the department. Her name was Nancy. However I pulled up right after her and got to go in with her.

The garage door was open with a car inside. The police that were there told us that the 'patient' was in the car in the driver's seat. We went in and Nancy reached in and placed her index and middle finger on the man's neck where the carotid pulse should be. There was none! At first she thought that we were going to need to pull him out and start CPR as his skin color was still good, which normally indicated that a person's heart had just recently stopped beating. However upon further evaluation, she noted that he was stone cold and also as hard as said stone. Rigidity is a definitive sign of death, meaning that he had been gone for a while.

As I said, I had never actually looked at a dead body before. Well... except at funerals, but those do not count because they have been made up to look natural. I will admit that as natural as this guy looked, there was the thought in the back of my head that this was a training run that was staged.

After we confirmed that he was deceased, the police officers explained to us that he was a husband and a father. It was his sister that had called asking for the police to check on him when he did not come to pick up the kids. She explained that his wife was sick in the hospital and that he had recently lost his job and he bills were piling up. He had made several statements about feeling worthless and depressed. His sister watched the kids during the day while he was looking for a job.

On this day he went home instead of picking up his kids and pulled into the garage and left the car running.

For those of you that do not understand, as I didn't back then either, a car puts out carbon monoxide from the exhaust. The blood cells in our body attach more easily to the oxygen molecule in that than to oxygen. It makes the skin turn a bright shade of red, but starves the body of the oxygen needed to live.

Over the years I have seen many suicides in many different ways, but this was my first. They are always sad and some, like this one, are tragic. So if you are reading this right now and you are someone that is feeling like death is the answer, I encourage you to please talk to someone before you make a choice that you cannot change. The thing that I have found to be most often true is that time has a way of making things better. Life is full of ups and downs. Don't miss out on the next up!

Gas Station Murder

It was a beautiful summer night. As was my custom on nights I did not work, I was doing a ride-along with my favorite city medic crew. They were in the heart of the city and were always the busiest truck as well. The night had been busy, but nothing truly exciting. Most of the calls city ambulances go on are simply sick people wanting a ride to the hospital and the occasional homeless person that is looking for a free meal and a place to sleep for a few hours.

Most of the 12 hour shift was over and it was beginning to calm down. Then the call came over the radio. "Medic 1 respond to the Marathon at the corner of .... You will be responding on a possible gunshot victim. Stage at the corner of ... and wait for police to arrive on-scene and clear you to proceed."

GUN SHOT VICTIM! These were the kind of calls that I lived for. My heart started to race as I got excited. The thrill of riding in an ambulance with lights and sirens blaring into the darkness of night is exhilarating and even better when I was on the way to an exciting kind of run.

We arrived at our dispatched staging area and waited, for what seemed like forever, for the police to hit us up on the radio that the scene was secured and safe to enter. As we pulled up to the gas station parking lot, there were more police cars there than I cared to count. The field supervisor for the medic crew arrived as well. It was not unusual for a supervisor to show up if it sounded like an extra hand might be needed, but on this night he also had a paramedic student riding with him that he thought might be able to get some experience.

As we exited the ambulance, several police officers approached us and one of them began telling us that the patient appears to be dead but they needed the medics to confirm that for legal coverage. The building was dark and old. Not only was it a gas station, it was also an auto repair shop with a single bay. A couple of officers led the way through the gas station as the two medics I worked with followed. The supervisor and the medic student followed and I took up the rear. We were led through the main customer area and into the repair bay into the back where the patient was found on the floor. One of the medics had taken in the heart monitor to confirm the death, but when they got inside they found that they did not need it. Rigor mortis had already settled in and that is a definitive sign of death. Since this was a crime scene, the goal is to disturb as little as necessary to preserve any and all possible evidence.

Having given their confirmation to the police detectives, we all turned about face and filed out of the station the same way we entered. Anti-climactic to say the least. However I did get to have my first experience with an active crime scene, which was pretty cool.

Now before you go thinking that this was the end of this rather boring story, let me teach you something that the medic student learned that particular evening. As we were standing around the ambulance chatting before we marked back in-service, one of the detectives approached us and pulled the supervisor to the side. After a brief conversation, he returned and told the student that he was going to have to leave with one of the police officers and go to the station and have his finger prints taken. It seems that as this student was meandering through the gas station, he was touching things. He was picking up things to look at them and set them back down and running his hands along edges of desks and counters. This left his finger prints ALL OVER the CRIME SCENE. This not only created a lot more work for the evidence tech, but it potentially destroyed other finger prints that might have been left by the actual perpetrator. Therefore he had to go down to the station to get his prints on file for them to be able to eliminate any prints he left behind.

Sadly I never did hear if that murder was ever solved. The media talked about the incident the day after it happened, but never followed up with the end result of the investigation. That is probably the case with most major crimes unless it is something high profile.

HIV and Head Injuries

Many years ago it was common practice to have nursing homes that were specifically for HIV/AIDS patients. This has changed due to increased patient privacy laws that said by placing a person in this kind of facility it was letting everyone know what medical condition they have.

While working on a Basic Life Support (BLS) truck one afternoon, we were sent to assist the local fire department with a head injury at the HIV/AIDS facility. When we arrived, we were met by a few of the fire fighters that explained that they were waiting for the patient to become unconscious. Apparently this patient had slipped on a wet floor and fell hitting his head. When he hit his head it caused it to split open and start bleeding. Head injuries bleed a lot due to the amount of blood that is sent up there. This particular patient did not want to live any longer and was insisting on being left alone until he 'bled out' and died. To keep first responders and nurses away he would whip his head around causing blood to fly towards anyone in the general area. The nursing staff referred to him as Jesus because he had long wavy hair and kind of resembled the image of Jesus in pictures. His long hair and all the blood coming from his head created a safety hazard. And he was spitting at everyone.

I, like many young people, felt invincible and would always take on the challenges presented before me. Not wanting to be out-witted by a patient and also to save the time of waiting until he passed out I went to the ambulance to take action. My partner unloaded the cot and a backboard while I got suited up. I put on all the infection safety gear we had; a gown, safety goggles, a hair net, gloves and a full face shield. I grabbed a hand full of 4x4 gauze pads and an oxygen mask and went in.

As I approached the patient he began whipping his head around sending blood flying my way and spitting at me with what saliva he could muster up. I walked up to him and placed the oxygen mask on his face to contain the spit as I knelt down onto his shoulders and chest to hold him down. Once I had better control of him I applied the gauze and my partner threw some kerlex my way to secure the gauze in place.

After having all the dangerous secretions contained, the fire guys and my partner came in to help me. We secured the patient to the backboard with straps and kerlex. This particular method of restraining a patient is now very much frowned upon, but was common practice back in those days. We then secured the backboard to the cot and got underway to the hospital.

The entire way, this guy fought and wiggled and writhed his way out of the restraints as much as possible. Ultimately I ended up straddling over him and holding him down for a majority of the trip. In between times when he would free himself from the restraint, I managed to call into the hospital (on the radio as cell phones were not a thing yet) and asked them to meet me with leather restraints and security. The rest of the trip consisted of just keeping the patient on the cot. After arriving at the hospital, we transferred him to their bed and they did apply better restraints until they could get him inside and sedate him with medicine.

After we were done and the truck was scrubbed

thoroughly with a heavy cleaner, I had to take a break and get some food. I do not think that I had worked that hard in a long time. Sometimes we have to make decisions and do things that could be considered harmful at times to prevent a patient from incurring even more harm and even death. I have said it before and will say it many more times, maybe this patient should have had the right to choose to die and not be forced to live with the disease he had, but that is not my choice to make and I am charged with always helping do what is in the best interest of a patient based on accepted medical standards.

He Loved Pussy Too Much

Sometimes when I worked nights and it got slow, we would go hang out in one of the major emergency rooms and talk to the staff and watch some of the exciting stuff that happened around us. It was during these times that I got to witness just how disturbed and depraved some of we humans can be. Please take heed and if you are an extreme animal lover, you should probably skip this story.

One summer evening my partner and I were lurking around one of the two busiest ERs in the city. I'm not sure where my partner went, but I was flirting with one of the cute nurses at the triage desk. We were chatting when a man walked up to the desk. He was kind of hunched over and looked to be quite distressed. He was wearing a trench coat with stood out as odd to us since it was a balmy night outside.

"I need to see a doctor please", the man stated in a subdued tone. The nurse replied by asking what it was he needed to be seen for.

"I JUST NEED TO SEE A DOCTOR NOW!" This time he was a little louder but did not want to draw any attention to himself. This drew concern from both of us for two reasons. First we didn't know what this man might have under the coat or in his pocket, and what he might be willing to do if we did not give him what he wanted. Second because someone this insistent had the potential for being hurt from some sort of criminal act and didn't want to draw attention to themselves.

The nurse was fairly seasoned in dealing with this kind of person and stood up and got stern right back. "Sir! I promise you will not see a doctor until I know what it is you need to be seen for. So you can either tell me or you can turn around and walk back out that door."

There was a pause from the man. It was plain that he was contemplating in his mind what he should do. Then we could both see that he clearly made a decision. Next he stood up straight, backed up from the desk just a little bit and opened his coat. What we saw took us both aback just a little bit. This man had a dead cat hanging from his penis. He quietly stated that it got stuck and he could not get it off and it caused intense pain when he tried to pull.

The nurse told him to close his coat back up and follow her immediately to the back. She took him back to a private room and immediately notified a doctor and security. When she returned to the triage desk, she told me that while it was a horrible sight to see, it was not the worst thing that she had seen in her time as a nurse.

I happened to be around later that evening and heard from the nurse that they were able to remove the cat without surgery and he was released into the custody of the local police to be booked for animal cruelty.

Is He Dead Yet?

In years past security was not so tight in the emergency rooms. It was not that uncommon for family members to be allowed to watch resuscitation attempts of loved ones in an attempt to provide closure that everything possible was done. This next story sounds completely crazy and unfathomable, especially to anyone that has been in a hospital in the last 10 years or so, but I assure you that it is true. While I was not one of the initial responders on this call, I was at the hospital when the finale happened. The beginning is being relayed as it was heard described by the first responders after this whole ordeal was completed.

The initial dispatch was for an unresponsive person. Upon arrival the patient's wife led EMS to the living room where the patient was found unresponsive. He was lying face down on the floor. Given his age, somewhere in his 50's, EMS assumed it was most likely a heart attack and proceeded to load the patient and get him to the emergency room as fast as possible. While EMS was working on the patient, they recalled the wife repeatedly asking if he was alive or dead. As they were focused on patient care, they stated that they kept repeating that they were doing their best.

When the ambulance arrived at the emergency room, they were immediately directed to the trauma/code room for the doctors to assess the patient and attempt to determine what was wrong with him. The wife had apparently followed the ambulance to the hospital as she arrived at the triage desk very shortly after the crew brought the patient inside. She was led back to the room where her husband was and placed just inside the door.

The staff was working frantically to figure out what had happened to the man so that they could start administering a proper treatment. The doctor asked the wife if she had any idea what happened leading up to his collapse. However the wife's only response was, "Is he dead yet?" The doctor responded with, "Ma'am, he is still alive and we are working hard to figure out what happened to him so that we can fix it. Can you please help us with any information?"

The wife stood there watching for a few more minutes, shaking her head and ignoring the doctor's request for information. After a few more minutes went by, she repeated her question. "IS HE DEAD YET?"

It was at this point that the doctor decided that she was not going to provide any useful information, so he again reassured her that he was not dead and then asked one of the staff members to escort her to a quiet room. However as the staff member moved to lead her out of the room, she stepped closer to the bed and pulled out a gun.

"Well if he ain't dead yet, then stand back!" she stated in a sharp loud voice. It seemed like a movie where everything kind of went in slow motion. Many of the staff looked up at the woman and saw the gun. They all started moving away from the bed, grabbing at the staff members that had not looked up. Just as everyone was away from the bedside...

BANG! BANG!

She placed two bullets directly into her husband's

head. Without any kind of remorse or emotion, she laid the gun down at the foot of the bed, took a step back and raised her hands on top of her head as she said, "Well he is now!"

It seemed like forever before security made it into the room and placed her in handcuffs. The staff stood against the walls still looking at each other in fear and disbelief.

The next few hours were chaos in the ER. The charge nurse had to immediately start requesting help from the nurses from other units and calling around to the off-duty nurses to see who could come in. The room had to be taped off until detectives could arrive and document the new crime scene. Hospital administrators were called in, as were chaplains and mental health staff to assist the ER staff that were in the room during the event.

Honestly I never heard what the outcome of her case was. She probably accepted a plea bargain as there was no media coverage of any hearing on this incident. However it was said in one article that she was a domestic abuse victim of decades of physical, mental and emotional abuse by her husband. I guess she just finally got tired of it and decided to take care of the problem herself.

Sometimes Nothing Goes Right

It was a late night for us. There were heavy storms all night and that usually brings out all the car wrecks. For some reason people seem to forget how to drive when the weather changes. On this particular night, the lives of several people were changed forever.

We were dispatched to the interstate for an overturned semi. While this kind of accident can be problematic for other drivers, it seldom causes any major injuries. So we climbed into the ambulance and started towards the exit that we were told was the site of the accident. Visibility was very low and we could not see very far up the road, so we were driving a little slower as we approached the area where it was supposed to have happened. We saw the flashing red and blue lights of the police car that was positioned behind an upright semi. We initially thought that the officer had just pulled the truck over. So we continued scanning the sides of the interstate looking for the 'dispatched' overturned big rig. Something of that size should not be that hard to   spot.

As we got closer to the tractor trailer that was 'pulled over', we saw it. Under the passenger side of the cab was a car. It was pushed into the muddy ground and partially crushed by the weight of the truck. My driver slammed on our breaks and swerved over to the exit, as we were on the other side of the interstate. As he was accelerating up the ramp to get to the other side, my heart rate went from about 80 beats per minute to roughly 200 beats per minute. This was the first accident this severe that I had responded to as a paramedic. In my slightly panicked state, I marked on the scene and requested a medical helicopter be dispatched to our location immediately. Not too long after I said the words, I realized that there would be no helicopter because of the severity of the weather. However, my comment on the radio caught the attention of the other ambulance in our area and they decided that we might need a little help and added themselves to the call. After a quick assessment of the scene, I cued up dispatch and requested that a heavy rescue fire unit be dispatched to our location for extrication. I was not sure if there was anyone alive inside or not, but I did not want any delay in case there was.

My partner and I jumped out of the truck and were met at the side of the car by the state trooper that was first on scene. We first went to the car and noted that the driver was under the front tire of the semi and he was deceased. However there was a passenger that was also trapped under the big tire and she was very much alive and conscious. I had my partner grab our medical bag and get a set of vital signs for me. Then I told the scared young lady that the fire department was on their way and we would get her out of the car as soon as possible.

While I was waiting for my partner to return, the trooper explained, from the statement from the truck driver, that the car had lost control on the wet pavement and swerved across all three lanes of the road, hit the guard wire on the other side and then slid back across the road coming to a stop 'in front of her rig'. He went on to explain that he had told the truck driver to stay in the truck as she obviously did not know that she had rolled on top of the car.

The fire department arrived on the scene and after getting a quick rundown of what had happened, they took over the task of moving the tractor off of the patient and prying the door open so that we could move her out. It was at this time that the trooper was asked to take the driver out of the truck. As he helped her down from the cab, she saw the car under the tires and she began to break down. He walked her to his car and after another trooper arrived, he took the truck's driver to the local emergency room where she received a sedative.

With the help of my partner, I attempted to start an IV so that I could give the patient some pain medication. However, I was not able to successfully get one started. Right after my third attempt, the other ambulance arrived and the paramedic from that truck was finally able to get IV access and we were able to help relieve some of the young lady's pain. Other than that, during the duration of the extrication, we just monitored her vital signs and helped keep her calm. We were all soaked to the skin as the rain never let up.

The fire department tried to use a large jack to lift the truck, but it was not tall enough. They switched to using extrication air bags. Those just pushed into the mud instead of lifting the truck. Each attempt was done with care and control as every movement of the truck's tire was hurting the patient. Finally, it was determined that the only possible way to lift the cab from the patient was to call in a special lift truck from a towing company. This proved to be no easy, or quick, task to accomplish. At this point in time, after having all but one lane of the interstate shut down, the traffic was backed up about five miles. The nearest lift truck was about 20 minutes away. So we just kept trying to reassure the patient and giving pain medicine as we could.

With the help of a state trooper leading the way and clearing the path, the boom truck arrived and took up position on the on ramp directly above the car. Due to the distance, the truck had to pull one side of the truck into the mud. When the first attempt was ready to be made to lift the truck, the tow truck started to tilt instead of lifting the cab. The concern with moving the truck back up onto the pavement was that the cable would be at more of an angle instead of straight up. This could cause the truck tire to be pulled towards the passenger instead of up off of her. After a quick but thorough assessment, it was decided that the risk had to be taken because there was no other reasonable alternative and the patient needed to be moved fast as she had been trapped for almost 90 minutes at this point.

So after thoroughly securing the truck and attaching the hook to the truck, I positioned myself in with the patient as they started to lift. As the tire started to come up, I immediately saw the crushed head of her fiancé between the tire and her leg. I motioned for them to stop lifting immediately and asked for a sheet or a blanket to 'protect her from debris'. I felt that she was being traumatized enough without having to witness the site that I had just seen. After covering her view, they lifted the tire up enough for us to get the patient out onto a backboard. After securing her to it, six of us began the treacherous climb up the muddy hill while trying not to drop her. It took a little longer than we would have liked, but she was safely transported to the truck.

With my EMT driving, myself and the crew from the other truck began the transport to the closest level one trauma center in the area. It was close to 30 minutes away in dry weather conditions. We worked as a team to cut away all of the patients wet and muddy clothing so that we could do a complete assessment of all the injuries she had sustained. We did our best to get her dry, cleaned up and warm by turning the heat up high. During our assessment, we determined that she most likely was suffering from a compartment syndrome from being crushed under the tire for so long. This is a condition that happens when a body part is void of any blood flow for an extended period of time, causing the breakdown of fat and muscle releasing toxins into the area. Then when blood flow is restored, those toxins get washed into the blood stream and cause a whole host of bad things to happen in other organs. We started two more large IVs and started to infuse boluses of normal saline.

I called report to the receiving hospital and we

continued to provide all the supportive care that we could during the trip. Upon arriving at the emergency room, we were met in the ambulance bay by the trauma team and they began their assessment on the walk to the trauma room. The patient was moved to their bed and report was given. Before we could complete our clean up and report, the patient had been rushed off to the CAT scan and then to emergency surgery.

Unfortunately I never did get much follow up on how she did, but I did hear from a friend of her family that she did well in the surgery and was home within a couple of months going through rehab. So while I may never know the total extent of her injuries, it was good to know that she was able to return home.

Drunk Drivers Suck

Over the years I have had the unfortunate task of responding to many accidents involving drunk drivers. More often than not, the person that is drunk is the one that walks away with the fewest injuries. Regardless of whether someone else is hurt or not, drunk drivers cause a lot of problems for the first responders and other drivers that get stuck in traffic backups. Especially in today's society with the ease of access to Uber and Lyft drivers, there is zero reason for anyone to ever drink and drive.

This was probably one of the most tragic accidents that I have had to respond to. Not just from what happened during the accident, but also because of the cause.

It was late, approximately 4 o'clock in the morning, when the call came in for a two car accident on the highway. There was a head-on collision between two vehicles, one was an SUV and the other a compact car. Apparently the driver of the SUV was drunk and had entered the highway going the opposite direction of the flow of traffic. A semi had noticed the truck coming the wrong way and slowed down considerably. However the car that was behind the semi had not seen the SUV and because she didn't want to slow down, she veered into the other lane just as the SUV was passing the semi and the two cars collided at a very high rate of speed. The driver of the car, a young woman on her way home from her first shift as a new nurse, died instantly from the engine of the car entering her chest cavity. The driver of the SUV, however, was still breathing when we went to check on him.

The fire department started extrication as we called dispatch to have a medical helicopter sent to our location. After the firefighters were able to pop open the door, we did our best to secure the cervical spine of the patient as we pulled him from the wreckage. The smell of alcohol was immediately noticeable. As we were pulling him out, it was obvious that his legs and pelvis were completely crushed. This is very concerning because of the amount of blood that can be accumulated in the pelvis and abdomen. Plus there are several major arteries in that area that can be cut open by broken bones.

We placed him on a backboard and immediately went to work getting his airway secured and two big IVs started to treat for shock. Intubating the patient was difficult because of the amount of blood going into his mouth, as well as the broken bones and teeth. I was just about to place a non-visualized airway in (not the preferred method, but used as a back-up) when the helicopter landed and the arriving nurse asked to have a chance to intubate. After she was successful in inserting the tube in his trachea, we looked at the heart monitor and noticed that he was is a dysrhythmia (a lethal heart rhythm), so we started CPR. After 15-20 minutes of efforts at reviving the patient, we decided to cease and pronounce him deceased.

This was a tragic accident that resulted in two lives being ended that early morning. At the time, none of us felt sorry for the drunk driver that had just killed an innocent young woman with his stupidity. However, in the days that followed as we heard more information, we found out the man that was driving the SUV was fairly well known in the county and was never known to be much of a drinker at all. On that particular evening, he had gone home after work and found a note from his wife telling him that she took their three kids and left the state and that he would never see any of them ever again. That is what spurred him to go out and get drunk. I am in no way trying to excuse his bad choices, but learning that information did make us all feel a little more compassion for him, feel a little guilty for having such evil thoughts about the 'drunk driver' and most of all feeling bad for the children that will never see their father again, even when they are older and can choose for themselves. Many peoples' lives were changed forever that night. It is my sincerest hope that everyone reading this will remember it when they are faced with the choice to drive after a few drinks and instead call a friend or an Uber/taxi.

Where Is The Blood Coming From?

Sometimes people are nuts. Sometimes people make stupid decision. This is a case of both.

I was working the 911 medic on this night and we were dispatched with a fire engine that was across the district. We didn't normally respond with this engine crew because it was in the response area of another truck. However on this night, that crew was out on another call. We were being sent out for what was called in as 'vaginal bleeding'. When we arrived the engine crew was already there and had gone into the apartment and started assessing the patient. My partner and I just brought in our cot for the patient.

As I walked in this is what I saw; One of the firefighters was talking to the patient's grandmother. The other 3 were gathered around the patient. She was an attractive girl that we found out was 21 years old. One firefighter was filling out a run report with the patient's information, another was getting a set of vital signs and the third was questioning the patient as to what was going on. Some   medics like to come in and immediately take over a scene and assume patient care. I, on the other hand, preferred to stand back, listen first and then to interject my questions later. My way of thinking, the other crew members need to keep their practice up too.

As she was questioned, I heard that the bleeding started about an hour ago, that it wasn't a lot but was concerning to her and that it should not be her menstrual cycle. All good information. Then one of the firefighters asked her what her social security number was. This is a very normal question, and sometimes young adults simply do not know it yet. However this particular lady stated, "You probably need to ask my grandma what it is. I have schizophrenia and bi-polar disorder and she is my legal guardian." It was at this point that I made the clear decision that we probably needed to just load her on the cot and get her to a hospital.

But... just before I could say that, she started talking again to the firefighter that was assessing her. "Sir. I am pretty sure that the blood is coming from my vagina, but I am not sure. It might be coming from my anus.

Would you please look and see if you can tell?"

In my head I am screaming "NOOOOOO!!!" Before that word could make it to my mouth, this guy blurts out, "Sure!" A case of a man thinking with the wrong head again. I am sure that he just heard her say she has schizophrenia. At this point I see all three of these guys' eyes popping out of their heads hoping to get a glimpse.

She looks around and then says, "Uhm. There are a lot of guys around. Can we go into the bathroom and you can look there?"

Whew... I thought surely this guy was smart enough to not go ALONE into the bathroom with a crazy girl and watch her take her pants down. Oh but I was wrong. Again he said, "Sure!"

Okay. Since I was apparently the only one that was thinking with the correct head, I was not going to let him go into a bathroom alone with her and have no witness to anything she might claim later. So I followed them. She walked in and dropped her pj bottoms and bent over and spread her butt cheeks wide open. She obviously had very little shyness.

The firefighter 'inspected' the area and told her that he could see some dried blood in the area but that he really couldn't say for sure where it was coming from. Case closed, right? Please know that I am laughing at you right now if you said yes.

This little lady was not satisfied with that answer and she proceeded to ask "would you stick your finger in my butt to see if you find any blood in there?" Yes she did. This time, however, I did not wait for him to say, "Sure!" I quickly interjected that was beyond our scope of evaluation in the field and a doctor would need to conduct that kind of an exam for her. He didn't seem happy with that answer, but he agreed with me.

Finally we got her loaded onto the cot and into the ambulance. She wanted to go to the county hospital so we headed that way. The whole way she kept begging me to start an IV on her saying that they were going to do it anyway and she wanted a paramedic to do it. I kept explaining to her that there was no indication for me to justify sticking her with a needle. Then it got real. She told me that they always have to get it in the little vein in the knuckle of her thumb. That is a classic sign of someone that seeks drugs. She just kept getting madder and madder at me because I was not giving her what she wanted.

We arrived at the emergency room and went to the triage desk. This is where everything came together in a nice pretty bow. The nurse that came over to us looked at the patient and said, "Weren't you just here last night?" To which the girl said she was. When I explained to the nurse why she was coming in, she looked at her again and said, "That was the same thing you were here for last night."

After having us place the patient in an observation bed, she informed us that she would be having one of the staff doctors come over right away because this girl had gotten an intern and a resident to stick their fingers in her anus the night before. I am not sure what ever became of her, but I have always wondered if she ever got another fireman to stick his finger in her 'butt' after that day.

Hidden Injuries

During paramedic school we, the students, have to complete many hours of precepted ambulance rides and clinical time in the emergency room. This combined with class room time, study time and regular everyday life can get to be difficult at times. However it does seem to differentiate those that really want a career as a paramedic and those that don't or that maybe can't handle the stress.

One of my ambulance days was with a fire department in a mid-sized city. I hesitate to say that they are out in the country, but they (and the hospital) are a little behind in the current medical practices. They were in fact great people to work with. There were just times that I, as a student, knew more than they did. It seemed like I was the one doing the teaching.

We were returning to the fire station from another call when we received a dispatch to respond to a multi-car accident. Upon arriving on the scene we found two vehicles that were involved in a T-bone collision. The story that we got was that the light was turning from green to yellow to red. When the light turned yellow the car in the right turn lane of the northbound side went to complete the turn to get out of the intersection and the other car that was in the southbound lane was accelerating in an attempt to get through the yellow. The result was that the turning car was T-boned on the driver's side door.

A fire engine had arrived first and was in the process of evaluating the patients in the vehicle with front end damage. We were assigned to the car with the driver's door damage. The passenger was able to exit the car without any issues and went with our EMT to get assessed as she was not complaining of any pain or injury. The driver was telling us that she was having chest pain where the door had been pushed into her. There was not very much intrusion into the car from the door, but there was enough that we were concerned about possible broken ribs. When the second engine arrived we requested them to come with the Jaws of Life tool and open her door. She was a little older and didn't feel comfortable trying to crawl over to the passenger side. It was a smaller car so we didn't feel that it would be beneficial to try to take her out the passenger side on a back board either. She didn't seem to be in any serious distress at the moment so waiting for the firefighters to pop the door open was acceptable.

Once the door was open we assisted the patient out of the car. She was not complaining of any severe pain at the time and there was no complaint of pain in her neck. Normally we would have placed someone in a car accident on a backboard, but when there is no tenderness in the neck upon exam we do not do the back board anymore. We sat her on the cot and buckled her in and loaded her into the ambulance. As I mentioned, she was older, in her 60's and a smoker. She had told us that she has a history of COPD (chronic obstructive pulmonary disease) and required oxygen sometimes. Therefore when she told us that she was starting to have a little difficulty breathing we placed some oxygen on her and she felt better. On the transport to the emergency room, the patient began to complain that the pain was starting to get a little worse and her mouth was beginning to get ashen in color. It was then that I told the driver to start the lights and sirens and put the patient on a non-rebreather mask to give her more oxygen. I was also able to get a decent IV started before we arrived at the ER too.

The emergency room that we took her to was busy because it was also flu season. There was only one doctor on duty and they were down 2 nurses and could not get any from the floor units to come down and help. When we arrived one nurse told us to go into the first shock room and someone would be with us shortly. Knowing that this patient was rapidly getting worse and that something serious was wrong we moved with urgency to get her into the hospital bed and get her on their oxygen. I waited for a nurse to give a report to as to the condition of the patient and to explain the urgency, but every one of them that walked by kept telling me to wait a minute, 'someone would be right with us'.

After about 5 minutes of waiting, I asked one of the crew to watch her as I went over to the doctor and pleaded my case for him to come in and evaluate her immediately. After hearing about her decline and how the accident happened, he didn't wait another second to follow me back to the room. The doctor immediately started to do a quick, but thorough, exam and did not like what he was finding.

Finally a nurse walked in to the room and asked for the patient report. The doctor told her before she took report from me that he wanted an x-ray tech to come stat and do a chest x-ray. When the nurse arrived I gave her a full report of what happened and how the patient had deteriorated quickly. She went to work drawing blood from the IV that I had started. Since I had handed over care of my patient, I went out to the nurses' station and started working on my run report. Especially in serious cases, I like to stay near the room to find out what all they find wrong as they get the results of their tests.

Shortly after she arrived, the nurse left the room to assist with another patient. The x-ray tech came into the room and needed help getting the x-ray board under her. I went in to help. It didn't take long at all for the doctor to realize that this patient had a tension hemothorax. Just for those who do not know, that is when one side of the chest is filling up with blood, thereby compressing the lung down making it very hard to breath and eventually can cause problems with the heart's ability to pump blood. By the time this was found, she was getting worse quickly. The doctor immediately started calling for a nurse to help. He wanted a medical helicopter called to transfer this patient to a major trauma facility and he needed to insert a tube into her chest to drain the blood so that she could breathe again.

I went looking for a nurse, but they all kept telling me that they were just too busy to help. Apparently those nasty flu symptoms trumped a patient that was literally dying from her injuries. Finally I was able to get the unit clerk to call for the helicopter and I found a nurse that would at least bring in the chest tube kit so that the doctor could start prepping to insert it. Fortunately I had some experience from the Navy that allowed me to assist the physician in placing the chest tube. There was no nurse to be found that was willing to come help the doc. So I helped him set up the kit and prep the patient. Together we did get the chest tube inserted into her and there was a lot of blood that drained from her chest. It didn't take long for this poor woman to be able to breathe better and for her color to improve.

While we were waiting on the helicopter to arrive, the doc asked for some fluid to be hung and attached to her IV site to help replace some of the volume lost with the blood. However when I went to do this, I found that the nurse had messed up the IV when she drew the blood. So I went about the task of trying to start another because she needed fluid and eventually a blood transfusion. After multiple attempts and no one else to try, I did find a good vein on her foot that I was able to get access to and start fluid replacement. That was the first and only time that I have ever started an IV in someone's foot.

Just as I finished starting the new IV, the helicopter crew arrived. As they were walking in they were asking who the nurse was for report. I quietly informed them that none of the nurses had really started care and that it was just me and the doc. I told them what I could and the doctor filled in the rest. One of the crew kind of whispered to me, "Sounds like we got here just in the nick of time, she needs to get out of here before they kill her". I just smiled and nodded in the affirmative.

I helped get the patient loaded onto the helicopter cot, finished my report for the ER and headed outside to watch them take off. It felt good to be able to jump in and help save a life, even at the emergency room.

Home Water Birth

In almost 25 years of working in EMS off and on, I can say that the one thing that I have never done is deliver a baby. Watching my son be born was a pretty amazing thing, but actually being on the receiving end of catching a newborn was not something that I have looked forward to. It is messy and slippery. This run was the closest that I have ever come to actually having to deliver a baby, and it was also a pretty scary one, at least to me.

Everyone at the firehouse had all been asleep for a while. The day had been pretty uneventful. Sometime around 2 a.m. the station tones went off waking us all up to dispatch us to a 'possible delivery'. We arrived at a town home apartment and were met by an excited husband. As he led us through the home and up the stairs, I noted many pictures hung on the wall of their 5 other children. These other kids were apparently staying with their grandparents for the weekend. There were toys and clothes spread all over the floors. This was a busy household.

Dad explained to us that they have been planning a home water birth with the help of a midwife. However the midwife was stuck in some traffic and was delayed in arriving, so they called 911 at the request of the midwife manager for us to be on stand-by just in case. As he was finishing this explanation, we were turning into the bedroom that contained a blow up Jacuzzi with mom sitting inside of it with water filled up to her chest. The water was warm, if I had guessed, I would have bet it was probably about 85-90 degrees. Our patient was wearing only a sports bra. She was prepared to give birth. The thing that stood out the most to me was the 'floater' that was in the water with her. For those of you that are reading this and have no experience with childbirth, let me explain what I mean. When a woman is getting ready to give birth, the baby's head puts pressure on the mothers intestines and sometimes pushes out a bit of feces. This is a normal part of childbirth but still not something that I was excited to deal with.

I asked one of the firefighters to get me a set of vital signs while my partner was gathering the patient's personal information for our run report. The midwife manager was on the phone and was requesting to speak with me. She began to explain how to go about doing a water birth. Having zero actual experience delivering a baby and even less training on water births, I was very uncomfortable with this undertaking. I explained to her that water births were not in my protocol or training and that for the safety of the baby and mother, that I would allow the baby to be born in the water but would have to immediately remove the infant to care for it instead of leaving it in the water as she was explaining to me. I told her that if she wanted it to go her way that she would need to get her employee here fast. Obviously I was making that statement for effect as this poor lady on the phone had no control over how fast her employee could arrive. Just as I was finishing this conversation up, the mother yelled out that the baby was crowning.

After handing the phone back to the father, I walked over to the hot tub with some urgency as I was putting on my gloves. Looking down into the water I could see the head of the baby starting to poke its way out of the mother's vaginal opening. Just as I was preparing to put my hands into the water to assist in the delivery I heard the midwife running down the hallway exclaiming, "I'M HERE! I'M HERE!" That was my signal to quickly move out of the way to allow the newly arrived midwife in to do her job. Just to add emphasis to this, I clapped my hands together twice and jumped backwards as I said, "I'm out!"

We hung around to watch the birth, partly out of curiosity and mostly to make sure that there were not complications that we would need to do an emergent transport to the hospital. Watching a water birth was a fascinating experience. The baby came out from the mother with relative ease and with very little assistance from the midwife. After the baby was free from the birth canal, it was brought to the surface and his little face was popped just out of the water for him to take his first breath in his new world. The water was perfect for cleaning the baby and he was given to his mother to hold while the midwife attended to the umbilical cord. Happily everything went perfectly as planned and we wished the parents well and departed back to our beds.

We thankfully got to sleep the rest of that night.

Don't Call the PoPo

It was a cold fall night. I was in paramedic school and working as an EMT for a private ambulance company. It was a somewhat slow night and so my partner and I decided to go sit in an alley between a couple of local night clubs. We sometimes enjoyed watching the drunks and talking with the women that would come up to us.

We had been there for a little bit when we watched a fire engine and one of the 911 ambulances drive up the street past us with their lights on. They slowed down to a crawl as they passed us. Then they shut off their lights and went up the street, turned around and drove back the other way. We thought it was a little odd, but not being able to hear the dispatch radio, we didn't know what was going on.

About 5 minutes later, one of the employees from a club came running up to us and told us that there was a man in the parking lot next to the club that had been stabbed. Things just got exciting. So we turned on our lights and rolled about 50 yards down to the parking lot where we saw about 5 or 6 guys carrying another man, who was limp, to one of the cars. I got out of the ambulance and asked if they needed help. One of the guys said that his friend had been stabbed in the club and one of them called 911 in the club but someone told him that they drove away. They decided that they were going to take him to the hospital in one of their cars.

My partner grabbed the cot from the truck and we put him in the ambulance and started to cut his shirt off and get a set of vital signs before we hauled ass to the hospital. He had been stabbed in the abdomen, but he was not bleeding much on the outside. I placed a bandage over the cut just to help absorb what little blood was coming out.

Just about the time when we were going to head off to the ER the 911 ambulance showed up and they asked if we needed help. The man was stabbed in the stomach and he was acting 'different'. Therefore it was an ALS (Advanced Life Support) type of run and they were the paramedic. So I told them what I knew and passed the patient off to them. They asked if we could just switch cots until they got the patient to the hospital and

I said we would meet them there.

So all-in-all this was not a very exciting incident. However I just want to point out that people do the dumbest things. One person called 911 while another didn't want the police involved, so they hid the location of the patient and decided they would take him by car. They were all pretty drunk, so one of them was going to drive their stabbed friend to the hospital and potentially kill everyone, plus potentially some innocent people. This type of thinking is the reason that we created the phrase, 'you can't fix stupid'.

You Won't Be Needing That Anymore

It was a slow night at the private ambulance service. My partner and I decided to hang out in the county hospital emergency room. We were standing around the main nurses' station when a police officer came walking in looking for a nurse. He explained to her that an ambulance was coming in with a very motion sensitive situation. They had driven the ambulance less than 20 miles an hour the entire way with a police escort.

As the ambulance crept into the ambulance bay, several firefighters approached the back doors to help gently retrieve the cot from the patient compartment. As the cot was pulled out, a very scared young man became visible and a sheet was covering him and something else that created a large lump. We did not get to hear what the officer had told the nurse, but we gathered it was very critical. The crew and the firefighters rolled the cot into the trauma room.

My partner and I, of course, followed the group of people that were anxious to see what this was. After all the nurses and doctors were in the trauma room the paramedic began to give report on what the situation was.

Apparently this poor man's wife had learned of her husband's infidelity in their marriage and decided that a little pay back was in order. Some of you may recall the Lorena Bobbitt incident that occurred many years ago. So she did not let on that she knew anything about his extra-marital affair and proceeded to slide down under the sheets to give her happy husband some oral sex. After he was good and happy, she decided that he didn't need that part of his body any longer and bit down and through the base of his penis.

It was at that moment, as the blood spewed out into her mouth, that apparently she had decided that perhaps she had made a mistake. She froze not knowing what to do. She was afraid to let go for fear that it might detach with her. So the husband managed to stretch across to the night table and grab the phone to call 911. Even after their arrival, she refused to unclench her teeth to release his member so they could bandage it up and get him to the hospital for treatment.

The paramedics did the only thing that they could think of which was to administer pain medicine to the husband and with the assistance of several firefighters, they slid the couple excruciatingly slowly over onto a backboard to get them onto a cot and to the ER. Ironically and possibly best for the husband, all the paramedics and firefighters were men, so they all took great pains to make sure they moved carefully.

After the medic had given the full report, the medical staff determined that it would be best to proceed with the couple initially left on the cot to prevent unnecessary movement. The nurses and doctors all got the supplies they felt they needed and moved into place. The lead doctor then told the wife that it was okay for her to let go of her bite so that they could start treating her husband. She refused and mumbled something inaudible. They attempted for about 5 minutes to convince her to let go of her bite on his penis, but all to no avail.

The couple of doctors that were in the room moved

off to the side, out of hearing of the couple, to discuss what they should do next. The only course of action that they all agreed would work would be to start an IV on the wife and paralyze her. This action would allow them to pry her jaws open and safely start treatment on the husband. They weighed the risks involved in doing this because when administering a paralytic drug, it paralyzes the patient's entire body, including their chest muscles that are used to breathe. They would have two patients to deal with at that point and would need to breathe for the wife until the paralytic wore off.

The doctors pulled a couple of nurses off to the side and filled them in on the plan. They told the wife that they were just going to give her a little sedative to help relieve some of her anxiety. This she agreed to allow preventing any fighting from her side. After the administration of the drugs, the wife became completely paralyzed and they were able to successfully open her jaw and move her onto another bed to treat her. The attending surgeon dressed the wound at the base of the penis and they rushed him to the operating room where a urologist was waiting to   help fix the injury.

I have often wondered what ever happened with that couple. Was the wife charged with any battery? Did they end up divorced or did they reconcile and forgive each other? These are the things that we as paramedics always wish we could know about our patients.

Listen to Your Doctor

Sometimes we in the medical field can only make assumptions about what has happened with our patients. However it is many times not very far off base when we presume that they did not pay attention to their physician as was probably the case in this story.

I was sitting around the firehouse studying when we got the dispatch to a residence for a possible cardiac arrest. We arrived at the same time as the fire engine crew and the family anxiously guided us to the bedroom where we found our patient. They explained that he had complained of being 'tired' and went to lie down. They did convey that he had a history of heart disease and high blood pressure and regularly takes nitroglycerin for chest pain. This was all indicative of a possible heart attack.

He was a 50-something year old man that was lying face down on the bed. We rolled him over and found that he was not breathing and did not have a pulse. Since CPR is virtually worthless when done on a mattress, we immediately moved him to the floor and began to do compressions. The bedroom that we were attempting to work in was very small and we could barely get 2-3 people in to treat him.

I called for the fire guys to grab a backboard and to have the cot ready so we could move him to the ambulance to continue resuscitating him. When we got to the truck we were able to get IV access and intubate while we delivered electrical shocks to the heart. There were a few times when we seemed to get a normal heart rhythm back on the heart monitor, but we never could get a pulse and his rhythm always went back into ventricular fibrillation.

After about 20-30 minutes of treatment on-scene, we got one of the firefighters to drive us to the hospital. We continued CPR the entire way without any improvement. Upon arrival at the ER, we moved him to a bed in the code room and we assisted the staff in their resuscitation efforts. There were multiple times when we thought we were making some headway as after nearly every shock he would convert back to a normal sinus rhythm (the normal electrical activity of the heart) but would rapidly decline back to a lethal rhythm. Ultimately after nearly an hour of effort, the doctor made the decision to call the time of death.

While we were cleaning up and finishing the run report we were outside by the ambulance. I don't know if the family knew we could hear them or not, but they were discussing the events leading up to their father's 'episode'. It seems that they happen to have left out that their mother and father had recently had sex that day. I overheard another family member say something about their father taking Viagra but not wanting anyone to know. No one was sure if he had taken the Viagra or even if he had used any of his nitroglycerin. The symptoms and the signs all suggest that he did in fact take both.

Viagra was initially being researched as a cardiac (heart) medicine that would replace nitroglycerin as a long acting vasodilator (opening the blood vessels up), however that use never panned out but they found one of the side effects was the current use today. The problem becomes that when you mix any of the erectile dysfunction drugs with nitroglycerin, it causes an irreversible drop in blood pressure. That would have caused the initial cardiac arrest and explained why we could get a temporary return of the normal heart rhythm without ever getting a pulse. The resulting drop in blood pressure would have made the blood volume too low to oxygenate the heart muscle.

My point in telling this story is to hopefully reach those that do not believe that mixing certain medications can be deadly. It most certainly is. Always listen to your physician and consult with your pharmacist before starting any new medication. They can check it against all your current medicines and find any potential cross reaction.

The Good and the Bad

Part of the job of an EMT and paramedic is to transport nursing home patients to doctor and other medical appointments. I have been in many nursing homes in my years as a paramedic and I have not found many that I would put someone I know in. This next story is really two in one. One story is funny and the other is not so much.

The entryway for this particular nursing home was the day room and dining room. My partner and I went in with our cot and sought out a nurse to find out more about our patient and get the paperwork. While we were talking to the nurse in charge, one of the patients started walking towards us. She was younger, maybe in her mid- to late-twenties. It was obvious that she had severe mental retardation which explained why she was in the facility.

"Hey you! You are sexy! Do you want some of this?" she kept saying. We looked at her and smiled and then went back to finishing up with the nurse. The patient kept walking our way. The   next time I looked over at her I noticed that she was unzipping her pants. The next thing I know her pants, all of them, were around her ankles. She then was just shuffling towards us as best she could with her pants down. She then started to work on her shirt.

I interrupted the nurse and said, "Uhm... Is that normal?" The nurse looked over to the now naked patient and said, "Yes. She does that all the time." The nurse shouted over to one of the aids to get the patient dressed and help her to her room. She acted so nonchalant about it. My partner and I were almost in tears laughing about the whole thing.

After the patient had been helped out of the day room, the nurse told us about how sad that patient's story is. Apparently they had had a male patient move into the nursing home a few months back that had AIDS. I told her that I knew who she was referring to as I had been on the crew that brought him in. Apparently a few days after he was moved into the facility, the young girl that had just 'propositioned' us had done the same thing to him. The difference is that he took her up on her offer. He found her room   one night after lights out and had sex with her. It was only one time, but he did his damage. He had transmitted the HIV virus to her and she now has to deal with all the stuff that comes with that disease.

The male patient was immediately transferred out of the facility into a lock-down unit that was primarily for dementia patients. The nurse told us that they were probably going to prosecute him for battery but the patient honestly didn't care because he was already dying and would never be put in a jail cell anyway. Sadly she is right because he would just infect other people in the jail with him.

We, as first responders, sometimes get to see the evils of this world in both emergency settings and outside of them. It does make doing our job harder at times because we know what evils seemingly normal people are capable of. We never know what someone might try to do to us in the back of our ambulances and thus have to always be on guard for the unexpected. That constant stress of the unknown sometimes comes home with us and we just hope that our families can be our strength during those times.

Bar Owner

On one cool Halloween night, I was working as a reserve for my local fire department on the medic truck. I was still an EMT and almost done with medic school. We were dispatched for an assault patient at one of the local bars. Fortunately there were several police already on the scene when we arrived because this was sometimes a rough biker bar.

As we walked through the bar to where our patient was, one of the waitresses was dressed up as a cop in a sexy cop uniform. I remember that because she winked at me and smiled. It is the little things that make someone feel good.

Anyway... we got to our patient and the police explained to us that it was the bar owner. There had apparently been a couple of patrons that were starting to fight and the owner got in between them to break up the fight. He was a big guy that seemed to have been in a fair amount of his own scraps and probably is normally able to stop the fighting pretty easily. This time, however, he took a fist to   the side of his head and got his bell rung. It didn't help that he was 'celebrating' Halloween pretty strongly himself. The alcohol smell emanating from him was strong enough to give us a contact buzz.

During our initial exam of him we didn't find any visible injuries, but his blood pressure was extremely high. This could have been normal for him and he just never bothers to have it checked, but it can also be a sign of a head injury. So we talked him into going to the hospital to get checked out, although it took a lot of prodding and discussion. Ultimately his 'woman' told him he was going and he said OK. He didn't want to be wheeled out of his own bar, so we let him walk out to the cot waiting by the ambulance.

As if dealing with a drunk biker/bar owner was not enough, he waited until we got all the way out there until he decided that he HAD to go pee. If we did not let him go pee, he was not going to go. So one of the officers and I walked with him into the bar and let him use the bathroom. Then we walked him back out to the cot. As we were getting him back onto the cot and started grabbing straps to seat belt him in, I happen to notice a glob of something drop from the side of the cot rail. Then the closer I started to look, I saw a lot of runny globs coming off the cot and leading to a trail that ran all the way back to the bar. Yup, you probably guessed it. Apparently he thought he had to fart, but it was not just a fart. He left a trail of poo from the bar to the cot and it was piled up on the sheet that he was sitting on. I was never so glad to be only an EMT on an ALS run in my life.

Finally we loaded him into the back of the truck and I started the drive to the emergency room. The ride started out fairly uneventful. However about half way there, I heard him start yelling at my partner and then I saw him taking a few swings at him. So I grabbed the radio and called dispatch, gave them our location and requested the police respond to assist with a combative patient. I pull into the median and went around to the back to help. Dealing with drunks was not new to me after working in a busy Naval Hospital emergency room before.

I climbed into the back and as the patient started to swing on my partner again, I grabbed the back of his hand and rotated it outward taking away his power. He tried to swing the other fist my way, but was met with me grabbing that hand the same way. Now I had him in a hold with both hands rotating outward. He was not happy. Now I was the bully that was hurting him, as he said. I told my partner to grab the kerlex and we secured his hands to the rails of the cot so that he could no longer fight.

Just as we were finishing securing the patient, the police pulled up behind us and came up to assist. We thanked them for coming, but told them that we were able to secure the patient and would be okay the rest of the way to the ER.

The rest of the trip was uneventful, thank goodness. We unloaded the patient into a room. While the medic wrote the run report, I got the lucky task of taking the cot apart and cleaning all of the feces off of it. My favorite thing in the world to do (insert sarcastic tone here).

Dealing with drunks I have always had no problems doing. Sometimes it can be entertaining and a little fun to mess with them. (Yes I know that I am evil for messing with drunk people.) But the one part of this job that I have never... ever... wanted to have anything to do with is dealing with people's poop.

Too Much Of a Good Thing

It was a beautiful sunny afternoon and I was happy to be hanging out with the fire department working as a reserve EMT. We were sitting out on the apron enjoying the sunshine when we were dispatched for an injured person. Usually injuries are simple basic level runs and so EMTs are normally the tech for them. When we arrived on the scene we saw a lady sitting on the ground in her back yard near a Koi pond. Assuming that I would be the tech, I jumped out of the truck and headed out to begin assessing the injury and getting the details while my paramedic grabbed the cot to bring to us.

About half way to the patient I saw it. There was bone visible from probably 25 yards away. I immediately stopped and yelled back for her to bring the trauma bag and a splint. Then I said with a grin on my face, "And by the way, this is your run now." She just stopped and looked up at me and her only reply was, "Compound?" I responded in the affirmative and headed back to the patient. This patient had broken both bones in her lower leg and they were sticking out of her skin.

This is known as a compound fracture in medical speak.

After making contact with the patient I began to remove her shoe and sock to check to see if she still had feeling and a pulse below the fracture site. If either one of those were gone I would need to move to straighten the leg back out to restore the pulse or the sensation or both. She explained to me that she had come down to the pond to catch a Koi to give to her neighbor for their pond. She had slipped on a rock and fallen, but her foot had gotten stuck between a couple of rocks causing it to break the bones. I noted a broken glass next to her, but she did not appear to be cut anywhere.

As I was finishing my assessment of her foot and ankle, one of the firemen from the rescue was coming down with a med kit. He moved to immediately start an IV and I noticed that he had Fentanyl with him that he was going to administer. Being in medic school I remembered that we were drilled repeatedly about getting a pain level from the patient before and after administration of pain medicine. It struck me because it dawned on me that she had not even really flinched while I was moving her foot around to remove her shoe and sock. When I asked her what her pain level was, she told me it was a zero, that she felt no pain. I asked her if there was any pain when I was moving her foot around. She stated that it was maybe a 1 when I was moving it.

"What was in that glass of yours anyway?" I asked.

"I was having a snifter of brandy to wash down my Xanax." she said with a smile.

Well that explained a lot. However I do not think that the rescue medic was paying much attention because he went ahead and administered the full dose of 100mcg of Fentanyl. Eh! I know she won't feel any pain now. We splinted her ankle in place and moved her to the cot.

Once we got in the ambulance, my medic partner told me to go ahead and start driving towards the hospital. As I was getting on the main road, I noticed in the rear view mirror that she was getting out more Fentanyl. So I got her attention and said, "Hey! By the way, her pain level was a ZERO before she got her FIRST dose of 100mcg back on scene." The medic replied with an, "OK!" Then she proceeded to give her another full dose. Who am I to question a medic? So I just drove as quickly as I could to the ER.

When we got into the ambulance bay, I helped pull the cot out of the back and then took up position at the head of the cot as we went inside. We had just gotten up to the triage desk and the medic was starting to talk to the nurse when one of the physicians came by. "This woman's lips are blue. Why are we not breathing for her?" he said in a kind of angry tone. The medic turned toward the patient and said that we needed Narcan. That is a drug to reverse opioid (pain medicine) overdoses.

The doctor stopped everyone. He told everyone to calm down and move her into a bed. We rolled her around the corner and moved her onto one of the ER beds and another nurse started to aid her breathing with a bag-valve-mask (BVM). The doc asked for a bottle of sterile water and a big IV needle. He took the needle and poked a hole in the top. He then used that to wash out the wound around the fracture site.

After he felt it was fairly clean, he took hold of her ankle and gently pulled down and re-aligned the bones. Just when he did that the patient virtually sat straight up in bed and screamed out in pain. Well, okay, I guess we didn't need to reverse the pain medicine. It was a good thing too, because once you administer Narcan any other opiate pain medicine (i.e. Fentanyl, Morphine, Dilaudid, etc.) will not work until the Narcan has worn off. And I am guessing she probably wanted the pain medicine after her leg was re-aligned.

I tell this story not because I wanted to call anyone out. Heaven knows I am sure I have made more than my share of mistakes when I thought I was acting in the patient's best interest. Also this particular medic is one of the best medics that I have had the distinct pleasure of working with. Rather I wanted to make a point that we all have different tolerance levels to pain and we all can use a reminder sometimes to actually listen to others even when we are busy and our minds are on other things.

The Abandoned Post Office

Working at the firehouse one cool evening we were called to go to an old post office building for an 'unconscious person'. The building had been a post office for years and years and was recently vacated. A local police officer had been patrolling in the morning of that day and saw a vehicle in the parking lot. This was not all that uncommon for him as he routinely saw cars parked there to talk on the phone, check their calendar, fill out some paperwork before going to an appointment, etc. It did catch his attention, however, when he drove back by the building about 8 hours later and the same car was sitting there in the same spot. So he pulled into the parking lot to see what was going on.

When he went up to the car to check on it he saw a young man in the driver's seat and when he knocked on the window there was no response. That is when he called us. When we arrived, we approached the vehicle and we did not get any response out of him either. As we started to walk around looking in the various windows, one of the firefighters noticed a pistol laying on the floor of the vehicle. That is when we also noted that there was dried blood on his nose. The young man was wearing a ball cap and that made it hard for us to see much else on his face.

At this point we knew that we needed to gain entry into the car, so the firefighters got their vehicle entry kit that allowed them to unlock car doors. During their process of unlocking the door, the engine officer made the decision that a couple of firefighters needed to get on their air tanks because it was recent news that people were killing him/her self with poisonous gas that would also harm or kill any first responders opening the vehicle to check on the person. There were also some people that were setting up explosive devices that were rigged to explode when the door was opened. So two firemen put on their gear and opened the driver's door while the rest of us stood several yards away.

After they did a thorough inspection, still being careful not to disturb any more than they needed to in case it became a murder scene, they did not find anything that would indicate any kind of poison or explosive devices. So we approached the car and did a quick assessment of the person inside. It was obvious that he had been deceased for several hours. Upon further exam, we found that he had indeed shot himself under the chin. His ball cap, although surprisingly still on his head, had covered up the exit wound that would have indicated his death from outside the car.

During our check of the vehicle, we found a note that was left by the victim. It read, "I have no family, no friends and no money. Good luck burying me. Goodbye!" Whenever I read things like that, I have to wonder if that was true or not. Did this person not have any family? Did he really not have any friends that cared about him? Or was that just what he perceived from a bout of severe depression. I will never know what the truth was about him or any of the other many suicides that I have had to respond to. What I will say is that virtually every single one of those people occupy my memory and they will never be forgotten by me.

He Died With a Smile

This is probably going to be one of those stories that some people will read and condemn me for being a hard-hearted ass and others will find it as funny as I did. The scenario itself was hilarious, the person's death and the effect on his surviving spouse was solemn and I did my best to recognize that and save her memories of her husband.

It was in the afternoon when my partner and I were sent out to a residence to check on an elderly person. The couple that lived in the home were in their 70's and so their neighbor checked up on them daily. On this particular afternoon, no one answered the house phone when he attempted to call and when he left work to go check on them, no one answered the door. Their car was still in the driveway and this gave the man cause to be concerned.

It was us, on the medic truck, a fire engine and a police officer that responded to the home. Generally before we start breaking into someone's home, we do a 360 degree check to see if   there are any windows or doors that are unlocked. We also go ahead and knock to see if anyone inside hears us. On this day, as one of the firemen knocked on the bedroom window the woman of the house opened the shades. She then came to the door and let us in. We explained to her why we were there. She told us that she had taken a pain pill that made her fall asleep and she did not hear any of the phone calls or door bells. She didn't know why her husband didn't answer though.

She gave us permission to check the house for him, as she was afraid to look around because of what she might find. She was right this time. The neighbor and I found her husband in his office chair. Upon checking him, I found that he was not breathing and did not have a heartbeat. Another quick check and I found that rigor mortis had set in and he was cold to the touch. This was an indication that he had been gone for a while. The neighbor told me that, while he was older, he had been a respected business professional for many years and he still did some consulting once in a while. This is what we assumed he had been doing in his office when he died.

After letting the wife know about her husband, we asked her if there was anyone she wanted to call to come be with her. We went ahead and let the engine crew go back in service and leave the scene. After she called some family to come. I explained to her that we needed to call his doctor and get their commitment to sign the death certificate, otherwise we would have to call the coroner to come and remove his body for the medical examiner to sign it. She did not know where the doctor's phone number was. She gave us permission to look around the house to see if we could find a prescription bottle or a business card with a name and phone number.

My partner and the wife started looking through the kitchen for something. The neighbor, the police officer and I all went into the office to see what we could find. While we were looking around, the neighbor had accidentally bumped into the mouse for the computer. This activated the screen that, up until then had been black. We were all a little taken back by what we saw. There on the screen was very vivid video of teen porn. As we looked, we noted that there was approximately

10 tabs open on the browser that all contained teen porn. While we looked at each other and tried to hold back our laughter, it all kind of dawned on us at once and we all looked down and saw that the man's little guy was hanging out of the zipper of his pants. He had died while masturbating. A seventy year old man was masturbating to teen porn when he died.

After we all got our little giggles out, the three of us decided that this was not a relevant fact that anyone else, especially his wife, needed to know. So we agreed to close out the browser completely and I, having gloves on, moved his member back in his pants and zipped them back up. No one but us needed to remember him in that way. While first responders do tend to find the things people do funny, most of us do really try to help people keep their dignity intact even after death.

Abusing the System

I was a fairly new paramedic and had started my first job working as one. I had worked as an EMT for many years, so I wasn't new to the ambulance though. This ambulance service was based in a hospital which was pretty cool because they used the paramedics as their Code Blue Team. We responded to all cardiac arrests throughout the hospital and they looked to us to run them.

While there were probably many patients that abused the 911 system, there was one that really stood out. She called 911 routinely several times a day unless her sister had picked her up for appointments. This woman was so bad that even her family didn't spend any more time with her than was necessary. Let me tell you about the day that I met her.

We were dispatched for chest pain. When we arrived I went inside to do my chest pain assessment. I did the full treatment. She got a full 12-lead EKG to look for a heart attack. She got baby aspirin and nitro. She got an IV started. Her little   apartment was very hard to maneuver around in and our cot would not fit back in the bedroom where she was. She had told me that she was blind and could not walk. So I got a couple of firemen and myself to carry her out through the apartment and to the cot. She gave me the full on description of having some kind of heart problem and so I treated her as such.

Then we got to the emergency room. EVERY SINGLE NURSE in the department knew her by name. I immediately knew by the look on their faces and their demeanor that I had just been taken. Sure enough I got the run down from one of the nurses. This lady was a regular in the emergency room and it was ALWAYS chest pain. The doctors did a full work up every time because they didn't want it to be that one time they didn't, to be the one that she was actually having a heart attack. So with every visit the doctors ordered a full set of blood tests and did multiple EKGs. Then they would call her sister to drive the hour it took from her sister's house to come pick her up.

This went on for a few weeks where I would occasionally be the medic that got the call and I would go pick her up. Never again did she get me to carry her large self to the cot. I found out she could see and walk just fine. She just didn't want to. Since we usually had two or three trucks in service, we all had our turn. And every time I took the doctor's advice and treated it just like a possible heart attack. At one point I asked why they didn't have a psychiatrist consult with her. They explained that she had been through all of that, but there wasn't much they could really do.

Then a day came when I had the good fortune of picking this lady up 5 times in a single day. She was apparently super bored that day and missed the company of the nursing staff. However I had come to my final straw when she called at 4 a.m. We got in the truck, I immediately disregarded the fire engine that was dispatched with us and we drove to her house. In hindsight, I probably handled this poorly but I was tired and had had enough of her crap that day. When we arrived, I told my partner to just stay put and I'd be right back. I walked into her house and told her to get her ass into my truck. She got right up and shuffled herself out and I made her climb up into the truck. I still had her sit on the cot and strapped her in. I told her that she was going down to the city this time to the county hospital. She said, "Okay". So I took that as consent and off we went.

I was taking her to the big city for two reasons. First so that hopefully she would not get home for a long while. Second because I was really hoping that they would be able to get her some assistance that the rural county hospital could not provide.

The 45 minute ride down to the city was uneventful. I mostly just watched her and wrote my run report. When we got to the ER we took her in to the triage desk. Remember that I was tired and cranky, but I decided that I was going to try to be nice to the nurses here and let them in on what was going on. So I explained to this triage nurse what was going on with the patient, her history and what I had hoped could be accomplished at their facility.

His response was less than helpful. "Wait. What? What county are you from? Why didn't you take her there? We don't do out of county psych here!" he said with his huffy attitude. He wanted to play a game, so fine. I can play it better than him. So I countered.

"Okay. Well she called tonight complaining of 10/10 chest pain radiating down her left arm with profuse sweating, nausea and dizziness. Now can you see her here?" I may have had a bit of a shitty smirk on my face. He looked at her and asked if she was having chest pain to which she looked at him and just shook her head yes. That was not what he wanted to hear, so he threw his pen across the desk and told me to hang on.

I think it should be said that this hospital can't legally tell me to take her someplace else anyway. They had to admit her and do an evaluation then transfer her out after they determined she was stable. But if he wanted to be snooty. I would give him a run for his money.

He returned with the charge nurse and I told her what all had transpired and how her nurse was being a real jerk. I heard her mumble to him that they cannot legally send her away once we entered her door regardless of why we came there. She turned back to me and finished checking us into the system and gave her a bed in the very back of the observation ward.

We proceeded to take her to her bed and moved her over with the assistance of her bedside nurse. I again gave her the rundown of what and why. She was much nicer and assured me that the patient would be there for quite a long while. Whew!

We finished up and headed back to station and I happily got to sleep the rest of that short night. The next morning I got a phone call from the fire chief asking why I disregarded the engine so fast last night on a chest pain call. I asked him why he didn't recognize the address, it was kind of a very distinct one. I explained to him about her pattern and that there was no need to keep the crew up for our 'favorite frequent flier'.

I never did get called to respond to her again. There were a few dispatches to that address, but none of them were for me. A few months went by when I got news that she had gotten admitted to one of the psych units down in the city. Somehow she managed to convince one of the doctors down there that she would be happier if she could have bariatric surgery AGAIN. Yes for the second time. However she died during the course of the surgery. I'll just leave that at that.

At Least He Had a Nice Rack

I have never been a fan of any kind for motorcycles. From a standpoint of the many accidents that I have worked with motorcycles involved, they are horrible. If the rider is lucky they get killed. However more often than not, they are left with debilitating injuries that affect the rest of their lives. Many times it is the rider's fault for not driving in a safe manner. It becomes way too easy for young riders to feel like they are small and much faster than cars so they can easily navigate traffic jams or get to their destination much faster. Even when the rider is doing their best to drive safe, they are just harder to see and in today's technological world where people are texting and surfing the web while driving, it is not always the rider's fault, but they are still the one that end up in the intensive care unit.

Many times after dropping a patient off in the trauma emergency rooms, we would hang out a little longer if there was something exciting on the way in. On this day the medical helicopter was landing with a motorcyclist that was in a wreck on a rural country road where it took almost 45 minutes for first responders to arrive. He was part of a group of riders that were cruising through the country side. He told the doctor that he was just riding along when a deer jumped out in front of him and he could not avoid the collision. Trying to be funny, the patient said, "Well at least he was a 12 pointer. I will have a good memento hanging on my wall after this is all done."

The man was in his mid- to late sixties, overweight and a diabetic. He was wearing his leather gear and his helmet. So his head was all intact. However the collision was such that he broke both lower legs in bi-lateral compound fractures. Part of the good side of his diabetes was that he had neuropathy in his lower legs, so the pain was dulled quite a bit due to a normal lack of feeling in his lower legs. The bad side of that is that his normal blood flow to those legs is severely diminished and that was going to cause a problem with them healing properly. After much discussion and many x-rays, the orthopedic doctor told the man that the only option that they had was to amputate both legs. If they tried to re-attach them, he had a high probability of getting a severe infection and dying.

This is why I personally will chose to never ride a motorcycle. It doesn't even have to be a car that does it to you. Nature will get you too.

Crying Wolf

Sometimes we in the medical profession have a hard time determining a patient's true intent. Many suicide attempts or threats are simply a cry for help. Sometimes it is just someone thinking that they are letting another person know where to find their body, but they take too long to do the deed and end up getting hauled off to the ER for evaluation and treatment. These next three cases I am including in a single chapter because I think that they show the differences.

Case #1

During medic school I was doing an overnight precepting shift in the ER. One of the city medics brought in this young man that had jumped from the fifth story window of his apartment complex. This was a pretty blatant attempt at killing himself and was not a simple cry for help. The only reason that he didn't actually die was because he landed on the grass that was very wet and soft from the recent rain that we had been having. He did however fracture several spinal vertebrae and lacerated his liver. So he came close.

The trauma staff got him fixed up and he spent three days in the psych unit talking with the psych staff. He told them how he had full-blown AIDS and that his family had disowned him because he came out as being gay. The final straw for him was when his boyfriend dumped him and moved out. He felt like he had no one and he was all alone. Somehow in that short three days of chit chatting, these psychologists felt they had cured him. I'm sure that he was feeding them all the right words and phrases because he just wanted to go home.

It was funny because I was on the crew that was taking him home when he was discharged from hospital three days later. He had a neck brace on that was screwed into his head that held his spinal fractures in line. He was on a few new medicines and was given instructions to simply follow up with his doctors the next day. Having been in the ER that night and hearing the story, I honestly felt very uncomfortable taking him home to be left alone. There was supposed to be someone meeting us at the house when we dropped him off, but they were running behind. He had a phone and family was supposedly on the way. We called our medical director, who told us to go ahead and leave him there. We called our company director and he told us to follow the doctors' orders and just document the heck out of this run. So we set him up at home, got his signature and left.

When we left, we went around the corner and listened to the city dispatch channel and sure enough about 30 minutes later there was a dispatch for a person falling from the building. This time, since his neck was already broken, he made sure that he landed on his head, on the sidewalk and he died on impact this time. That was a case of someone that was going to fulfill his intentions whether it was then or a week later or a month later.

Case #2

The next story happened when I was working at a rural hospital ambulance service. The local police brought in a young girl that had told a friend that she was going to die because she just hated living. When the ER doc evaluated her, she admitted to saying it but that she was just in a 'mood' and wanted to see who cared. She really wasn't acting like she was depressed or in distress. So the doctor decided that she was fine and didn't need a sitter to be with her to make sure she didn't do anything stupid. Well that was his first mistake.

As soon as she took note that no one was watching her, she peeked out the door and found the exit and she took off running at full stride out the door. The ER staff went chasing after her and she ran straight into the pond across the parking lot. She tried to swim to the other side, but the pond was quickly surrounded by security and medical staff. She eventually got too cold (it was a cool fall day) and came out. They marched her back into the ER, gave her some scrubs so that she could get out of her wet clothing and she had bought herself a babysitter, i.e. a security guard, to watch her until we could transfer her to the psych hospital for evaluation and treatment.

That is when I come into the picture. I drew the proverbial short straw and it was my turn to take the next run. After I heard that whole story, I asked her if she was going to give me any problems or if we could do this the polite way. She told me that she promises that she will not give me any trouble and she would prefer to walk. I explained to her that if I had to chase her, she would be going to the other hospital in chains.

I gathered all of my paperwork and was ready to head out. A security guard was coming along because of the problems that she had been already. So he was walking in front on the way out to the ambulance. The patient went next and I took up the rear. Everything seemed to be going smooth. That is until she noticed the exit door out of the ambulance bay. She thought she was going to be slick and just started to veer off towards that direction. She didn't try to run, so I am not sure if she was just testing to see if I was paying attention or not. I saw her looking and knew she was going to try it, so I was ready. The minute she took one step off the proper path, I had my hands on her shoulders redirecting her and reminding her that I would put her in chains if she did that again.

We got into the ambulance and put her

onto the cot. We are supposed to place all three straps and two shoulder straps on every patient. However most of the time we only do two or three of the straps. This time I put her in the full seat belt system. We got on our way and for quite a while it didn't seem like I was going to have any issues. As soon as she thought I wasn't paying attention again, I saw her little fingers creeping towards the seat belt latches. I let her get one undone and I wanted to see how slick she really thought she was. After she managed to creep to the second, she made a bee line for the third. It didn't take me but a second to be right on her to keep her from getting up and re-secure her.

I told her that if she did that again, I would watch her jump out an ambulance that was traveling about 80 mph down the interstate. I told her if she hit just right, maybe she would die. I said that however if she didn't hit the pavement just right, she would roll and tumble probably get run over by other vehicles causing bones to break and skin to rip and tear. I said it might be a while before she hit her head and unconsciousness was hit or miss. So she was taking a huge risk of being in an immense amount of pain and getting to spend a few months in an ICU. Her eyes got big as saucers, but I didn't have another issue out of her. And besides the security guard got a good laugh.

She was one of those cases where I don't think she really wanted to die, but she was ready to take some pretty big risks that could have very well killed her just to see who would pay attention to her. So even if you think someone is crying wolf, you never know what they might have planned that will actually end up killing them anyway. Which leads me to the final case in this chapter.

Case #3

This happened while I was working in an emergency room. A girl was brought into our facility complaining of severe abdominal pains. She had been throwing up violently for the last hour.

As it turned out she had a boyfriend break up with her a few nights earlier and she got mad and was going to make him sorry by pretending to kill herself. She took an entire brand new bottle of Tylenol. When all was said and done, the boyfriend left and she stormed off to bed to cry. She told us that she didn't think that anything would come of it as it was 'just' Tylenol. What she failed to understand is that a Tylenol overdose is extremely lethal, it just takes a couple of days for the medicine to kill the liver.

A few days had passed and she had moved on. However the Tylenol was strong at work killing off her liver, and in effect killing her. By the time she actually came into the emergency room, the damage had been done and there was nothing that could possibly be done for her. It was one of the hardest things that the ER staff has ever had to do. They had to tell the family to call everyone in to say their final goodbyes because she wasn't going to live much longer. She was 17 years old and going to die from a stupid mistake pretending to commit suicide.

They gave her pain meds to help with the pain in her stomach. After she said all of her goodbyes, the doctors induced a coma to make her final hours pain free. She was moved up to   the ICU where over the next few hours her clotting factors disappeared. She started to bleed from her ears, eyes and any other hole in her body. Once the blood started to leak out it didn't take very long for her to die.

So again, crying wolf is sometimes a very deadly game that people play. Please always take heed when someone says they are going to kill their self. Even if they don't really mean it, if they are not careful they could kill themselves by complete accident.

Paramedic Lingo

This is NOT an exhaustive list of the words and sayings that paramedics/EMTs use. These are just a few that came to mind as I wrote this book that might give the reader some insight next time they are listening in to a conversation. Different regions may use different sayings.

Working a code – cardiac arrest

Code Brown – the patient pooped in their pants

Code Yellow – the patient urinated in their pants

10-0 – the patient is deceased

Running Hot – driving with lights and sirens on

CCFCP – Coo Coo For Coco Puffs (Crazy)

FDGB – Fall Down Go Boom (Fell down)

STEMI – Is a form of heart attack that is found after evaluating an EKG.

EKG – Is an print out of the electrical activity of the heart.

BLS – Basic Life Support. This consists of mostly minor injuries, common sickness and uncomplicated births.

ALS – Advanced Life Support. This requires a paramedic or higher and consists of anything requiring IVs, EKGs or most medications.

C-spine the patient – This means that we applied a C-collar around the neck and placed the patient on a backboard to protect against a possible broken neck.

MVA/MVC – Motor Vehicle Accident/Crash

Tube – The act of placing a tube in the patients throat to provide a secured way to breath for them.

Road Muffin – This is what we refer to motorcyclists that choose not to wear proper head protection, and/or that wear shorts and tank tops.

Blow Fluids – This is the act of infusing a large

amount of IV fluids in patients that are in a state of shock.

Compound Fracture – This is a broken bone that had broken the skin. Often thought of as having bone sticking out of the skin, but that is not always the case.

Defibrillate – In an attempt to 'reset' the heart during a cardiac arrest we deliver a shock of electricity to the heart.

ETOH – drunk or smells like alcohol

Bari/Bariatric – an obese patient that is too large to fit on a regular cot/bed.

Gold Card – Medicaid card

DOA – Dead On Arrival

Frequent Flier – A person that calls 911 frequently. Usually for things that do not require an ambulance.

Seeker – A patient that makes up complaints in the

sole attempt to get pain medicine due to an addiction.

Pneumo/Tension Pneumo – This a condition where air or blood gets between the chest wall and the lungs compressing the lung(s) down making it hard to breath.

A Stick – Commonly used to refer to an attempt, successful or not, to start an IV.

Vitals – This refers to taking the pulse, blood pressure, EKG, temperature, etc. Not all of these are taken every time.

Rig – ambulance

Tech – the person that provides patient care in the back while the other person drives. Can be used as a noun or a verb.